TAI CHI
FOR BALANCE

Simple Chair-Based Exercises For Injury Prevention, Enhanced Mobility,Strength,Flexibility, And Wellbeing

(For Beginners And Seniors)

JIANMING WONG

TABLE OF CONTENTS

INTRODUCTION

Tai Chi, also known as Tai Chi Chuan, is a traditional Chinese martial technique that has developed into an elegant form of exercise and meditation. Tai Chi, rooted in ancient Chinese philosophy, blends gentle, flowing motions with deep breathing and awareness. The practice focuses on balance, coordination, and the development of vital life force, known as "qi" or "chi."

Choreographed motions, often known as forms or sets, are designed to encourage the free flow of energy throughout the body. Tai Chi is more than simply a physical exercise; it is a holistic discipline involving the mind, body, and spirit.

Who Can Practice Tai Chi?

Tai Chi is an accessible and flexible practice for individuals of all ages and fitness levels. Its soft nature makes it ideal for anyone with physical limitations or health issues. Who can benefit from doing Tai Chi?

Seniors: Tai Chi is well-known for boosting balance, flexibility, and joint health, making it an ideal exercise for seniors looking to maintain or enhance general health.

People With Limited Mobility: Seated Tai Chi versions are available, enabling those with mobility limitations to benefit from this art form while sitting in a chair.

Beginners: Tai Chi has a progressive learning curve, making it ideal for novices. Tai Chi's advantages do not need any previous martial arts or fitness training.

Tai Chi, with its slow, methodical motions and concentrated breathing, is an excellent stress-relieving technique. It relaxes the mind and reduces general stress.

Those Seeking Mind-Body link: Tai Chi emphasizes the link between the mind and body. It encourages self-reflection, awareness, and a healthy balance of mental and physical well-being.

Athletes and fitness enthusiasts may use Tai Chi to enhance their balance, flexibility, and total body awareness.

Anyone Interested In Holistic Wellness

Tai Chi is a low-impact workout that helps relieve stress and improve general health.

Tai Chi is a practice that is accessible to anybody looking for a peaceful, contemplative, and comprehensive approach to physical and mental wellness.

The Essence Of Seated Tai Chi

Take a trip into the Zen Zone, where sitting Tai Chi transforms the ordinary into exceptional. Learn how to use moderate, sitting motions to create a tapestry of peace, restoring balance to

your mind and body without leaving
your chair. It's not simply a sitting
exercise; it's a way to calm.

IMPROVE YOUR HEALTH ONE SITTING MOTION AT A TIME

Discover the calm world of seated Tai Chi, a gentle and transforming approach to this age-old practice intended specifically for those who want to remain comfortably seated while reaping the benefits.

Do the flowing motions in ancient Tai Chi forms remain a mystery better left unsolved, or are the forms too taxing, like walking a tightrope? You could be a great candidate for seated Tai Chi. It makes Tai Chi more accessible to everyone, like experiencing its beauty while cuddled up in your favorite chair.

This new Tai Chi technique is ideal for the elderly, those with restricted mobility, and anybody searching for a mindful workout that does not need standing. Say goodbye to fears about being imbalanced while executing difficult motions; your chair will be your trustworthy friend!

There are several perks. Tai chi while sitting may enhance strength, flexibility, balance, and provide a profound sensation of relaxation. It's ideal for elders since it offers a gentle but effective way to maintain energy and well-being.

The opportunities for practicing Seated Tai Chi are limitless. When practicing Tai Chi, your chair may become your own refuge, whether you're in a community center, at home, or even at work (just imagine how quiet it can be during a hectic workday!).

What differentiates seated Tai Chi? It all boils down to posture elegance, movement flow, and the ability to breathe mindfully. Imagine yourself floating on a cloud while you focus on achieving inner harmony. Your chair is a continuous friend, providing the support and stability you need to thrive.

Tai Chi provides several benefits that are especially important to the senior population.

Improved Balance And Stability
One of Tai Chi's most well-known benefits for seniors is its remarkable ability to improve stability and balance. These essential components of movement usually degrade with aging, increasing the risk of falls and

injury. Tai Chi's slow, methodical motions, paired with its focus on posture and weight shifting, may help seniors build stronger legs and core muscles, increasing stability and confidence when moving.

Reduced Risk Of Falls

Falls are a significant source of worry for older persons because they often result in serious injuries and loss of independence. Tai Chi's focus on balance and coordination has been shown to drastically reduce the incidence of falling among seniors. Seniors who practice Tai Chi on a regular basis may lower their risk of falling both inside and outdoors by improving their proprioception (knowledge of their body's posture) and response time.

Improved Joint Health And Flexibility

Aging may induce stiffness and decreased flexibility, making regular chores more challenging. Tai chi's smooth, flowing movements increase flexibility, lubricate joints, and reduce stiffness. Seniors who practice on a daily basis may benefit from enhanced mobility and reduced joint discomfort, making it simpler for them to live active lifestyles.

De-stressing And Mental Health

Stress and anxiety are typical problems for individuals of all ages, even seniors, in today's fast-paced world. Tai Chi allows seniors to quiet their thoughts and cultivate inner serenity, providing a refuge of calm in the midst of stress. Tai Chi's careful, slow movements reduce stress, improve mental health, and promote relaxation. Seniors may find solace in the present moment by practicing Tai Chi, which has a meditation component that encourages attention and presence.

Improved cardiovascular health.
Tai Chi is gentle on the joints, yet it provides a lot of benefits for the heart. Tai Chi's slow and regular motions strengthen the heart, lower blood pressure, and enhance circulation. Regular Tai Chi practice may help seniors improve their cardiovascular system and reduce their risk of heart disease and stroke.

CHAPTER 1

CREATING YOUR PRACTICE SPACE

Creating an appropriate practice environment is crucial for seniors to receive the full advantages of Tai Chi, particularly when practicing seated Tai Chi for fall prevention. A well-prepared setting not only improves safety, but it also encourages calm and concentration.

Choose The Right Location

Quiet and Calm Environment

Choose a spot in your house that is free of distractions and noise. This will allow you to concentrate and completely participate in the motions.

Ensure that your arms and legs can move freely. While sitting Tai Chi occupies less space than standing routines,

Stable Chair

Select a robust chair without wheels. A chair with a backrest provides support, while armrests might improve stability while getting in and out of the chair.

Place your chair on a nonslip mat or rug to prevent it from moving while you exercise. Avoid using a chair on a slippery floor unless it is correctly positioned.

Remove any obstructions, such as furniture or loose carpets, that might cause a trip or fall.

Pleasant Seating

Select a chair that is pleasant to sit in for long amounts of time. It should provide enough back support while also allowing your feet to rest flat on the floor.

Proper Lighting: Keep the area well-lit to avoid eye strain and create a safe atmosphere.

Ventilation: Proper airflow maintains a suitable temperature and offers fresh air, which improves relaxation and focus.
To create a relaxing environment, decorate the place with soothing features such as plants, mild lighting, or soft hues.

Ambient Sound: Use gentle, contemplative music or natural noises to help you relax and concentrate throughout your practice.

Supportive Props: Keep a few pillows or cushions on available to help support your back or feet if needed.

Hydration: Keep a bottle of water available to remain hydrated, particularly if you intend to practice for a long time.
teaching resources: Keep books, movies, and other teaching resources within easy reach. A tablet or laptop may be used to study Tai Chi lessons or online sessions.

Pre-Practice Routine: Create a routine that marks the start of your practice. This may be lighting a candle, taking slow breaths, or doing mild stretches.

Warm-Up Area: Set aside a small area for warm-up activities before starting your Tai Chi practice. Gentle stretching or gentle exercises might help prepare your body and mind for the session.
Maintaining a clean and clutter-free practice room will help to create a good and welcoming environment.
Periodic Checks: To maintain continued safety, examine your chair and surrounding environment for signs of wear and tear or possible risks.

UNDERSTANDING YOUR BODY'S ALIGNMENT

Proper body alignment is an essential component of Tai Chi, especially for seniors who practice it sitting. Understanding and maintaining proper alignment may help avoid injuries, improve balance, and increase the overall efficacy of your actions.

Feet Placement
Keep your feet level on the ground, shoulder-width apart. This offers a sturdy basis and helps to distribute your weight evenly.

Kneeling Position: Keep your knees aligned with your feet. Avoid having them collapse inward or spread outward. Your knees should be just above your ankles to ensure good leg alignment.

Sit Upright: Keep your back straight and sit tall. Do not slump or lean too far forward or backward.

Place your pelvis in neutral alignment. This indicates that your lower back should be naturally curved, rather than abnormally arched or flat.

Distribute your weight equally over both sit bones. This equilibrium eliminates unneeded effort on one side of your body.

Upper Body: Spine And Shoulders

Spine lengthening

Imagine a cord slowly tugging the top of your head to the ceiling, lengthening your spine. This vision promotes a tall, upright posture.

Your shoulders should be relaxed and low, not hunched up to your ears. This relaxation relieves stress and improves breathing.

Head And Neck Alignment

Head Position: Keep your head in line with your spine. Your chin should be slightly tucked, forming a straight line from the top of your head down your spine.

Look straight ahead with a kind glance.
Avoid tilting your head too much up or
down.

Arm And Hand Positioning

Natural Curve: Allow your arms to hang
naturally at your sides, with a small bend at
the elbow. This stance promotes smooth Tai
Chi motions.
When moving your hands and arms, make
sure your wrists, elbows, and shoulders are
in a comfortable, natural position. Avoid
locking your joints.

Deep Breaths: Take deep, diaphragmatic
breaths. This entails breathing deeply into
your abdomen, allowing it to expand as you
inhale and constrict when you exhale.
Maintain a mild activation of the abdominal
muscles. This core engagement strengthens
your spine and aids with balance and
stability.

Awareness: Throughout your practice, keep your body in harmony. Check your posture on a regular basis and make any necessary modifications.

Perform a mental scan of your whole body, from head to toe, to ensure that everything is in alignment and relaxed. This scanning approach promotes optimal alignment and strengthens your mind-body connection.

Regular Adjustments

Don't be scared to make little tweaks throughout your practice. Even modest adjustments may greatly enhance your alignment and comfort.

Use props such as cushions or pillows to help you maintain your posture. For example, putting a cushion behind your lower back may assist to retain your spine's natural curvature.

Daily Routine

Include alignment checks in your everyday routine, not only during Tai Chi practice.

This practice helps you maintain healthy
posture and alignment throughout the day.

CHAPTER 2

BREATHING TECHNIQUES FOR RELAXATION AND ENERGY

In Tai Chi, breathing is far more than a physical action—it is a profound tool for cultivating energy (Qi), promoting relaxation, and boosting vitality. Mastering the art of intentional, mindful breathing can harmonize the body and mind, creating an inner equilibrium that enhances overall well-being. Proper breathing supports the flow of Qi, the body's vital life force, enriching both physical and mental health.

One of the foundational practices in Tai Chi is diaphragmatic breathing—a deep, abdominal style of breathing that maximizes the efficiency of the breath. This technique encourages the full expansion of the lungs, fostering better oxygen exchange and a more profound sense of calm and energy.

To begin, place one hand on your abdomen and the other on your chest. As you inhale deeply through your nose, allow your abdomen to gently expand outward, feeling the air fill your lower lungs first. On the exhale, release the breath slowly through your mouth, allowing your abdomen to contract inward. This rhythmic, deep breathing activates the parasympathetic nervous system, promoting relaxation and focus.

In Tai Chi, breathing isn't just about the inhale and exhale—it's about the seamless connection between breath and movement. Each breath should flow in harmony with the fluid, graceful motions of Tai Chi, with inhalations linked to expansion and exhalations tied to release. This synchronized pattern of breathing helps to regulate the flow of Qi, fostering energy, clarity, and peace while also enhancing physical endurance.

Another key technique in Tai Chi breathing is reverse breathing. This practice involves consciously drawing in the abdomen during exhalation and expanding it during inhalation. While this may feel counterintuitive at first, reverse breathing is thought to stimulate deeper Qi circulation, optimize energy flow, and activate the body's natural healing processes. To practice, breathe in deeply through your nose, allowing the abdomen to expand outward. Then, as you exhale, gently draw your abdomen in toward your spine, pressing the breath out with focused intention.

Incorporating these breathing techniques into your Tai Chi practice provides a powerful means of relaxation, energy cultivation, and vitality enhancement. Whether you are facing the stresses of daily life or simply seeking greater clarity and strength, the mindful practice of deep, rhythmic breathing offers a path to inner peace and physical resilience.

Grounding And Centering Practices In Tai Chi For Seniors

For seniors, maintaining a sense of balance, stability, and mental clarity is essential, both in Tai Chi practice and in daily life. Tai Chi's grounding and centering exercises offer an invaluable method to achieve these goals, promoting physical equilibrium, mental calm, and overall vitality.

At the core of these practices is the principle of grounding—connecting deeply with the earth beneath you to cultivate a sense of stability and rootedness. To begin, stand with your feet shoulder-width apart, knees slightly bent, and your body relaxed. Imagine your feet as roots extending into the earth, anchoring you to the ground. As you breathe deeply and slowly, focus on the sensation of your feet connecting with the floor, drawing energy from the earth to center yourself.

Centering in Tai Chi refers to aligning your body's energy and focus with your core, or "dantian"—an area located just below the navel. By focusing on this point of inner strength, you bring your awareness to the center of your body, promoting balance and fluidity in both movement and thought. While standing or moving through Tai Chi forms, concentrate on this core center, breathing deeply and steadily to enhance your sense of stability and focus.

These grounding and centering exercises provide seniors with the tools to foster a deep sense of inner balance, both physically and emotionally. They help improve posture, enhance flexibility, and prevent falls while also cultivating mental clarity and emotional calm. By incorporating these practices into a regular Tai Chi routine, seniors can improve their resilience, energy levels, and overall quality of life.

Gentle Wind Chimes (Stand or Sit). Stand with feet shoulder-width apart and slightly bent knees, or sit comfortably in a chair with feet flat on the ground. If you feel at ease, gently close your eyes.
Inhale slowly and deeply via your nose. While exhaling, imagine your body as a collection of wind chimes. Sway your torso side to side, causing a mild twisting sensation in your spine. Breathe slowly and naturally as you

move. After a few sways, exhale to
return to center.

**Feeling The Breath (standing or
sitting)**

Stand shoulder-width apart with
slightly bent knees, or sit comfortably
on a chair, feet flat on the ground. Put
one hand on your tummy, and the other
hand on your chest.
Take a slow, deep inhalation through
your nose. Inhale and feel your
stomach expand. Your chest may lift
somewhat.Exhale slowly through your
lips, feeling your stomach constrict.
Continue to breathe deeply for a few
cycles, focusing on the sensation of air
going through your body.

Qigong Tennis Ball (Seated)

Sit comfortably in a chair, feet flat on the floor and back straight. Hold a tennis ball or comparable object in your palms and place it comfortably in front of your lower abdomen. Concentrate on your breathing, inhaling slowly and expelling completely.

Inhale, extend your belly, and gently press the ball outward. Exhale, imagine pulling the ball back towards your navel. Continue to take a few breaths, focusing on the interaction between your breath and the movement of the ball.

Mindful Breathing (3 Mins) Begin by finding a comfortable sitting or standing position. Close your eyes and take several deep breaths, concentrating on the sensation of air entering and exiting your body. With each inhalation, imagine drawing energy from the earth beneath you. As you exhale, imagine releasing tension and stress, allowing yourself to feel more grounded and centered.

Rooting Exercise (3 Mins)
Stand with your feet shoulder-width apart, knees slightly bent, and arms relaxed by your sides. Imagine roots growing from the soles of your feet deep into the ground, firmly anchoring you in place. Shift your weight slightly forward and backward, side to side, and in circular motions to feel the connection between your feet and the ground below you. This exercise promotes balance and stability.

Body Scan Meditation (3-5min) Sit or lie down in a comfortable position. Close your eyes and focus your attention on each part of your body, beginning with your toes and gradually moving up to the crown of your head. Identify any points of tension or discomfort and consciously release them with each exhale. This practice relaxes and centers the mind and body.

Tai Chi Ball Visualization (5-minute)
Stand shoulder-width apart, knees slightly bent. Consider holding a large, heavy ball in your hands at chest level. As you inhale, imagine drawing the ball inward toward your body and feeling energy gather in your center. As you exhale, imagine pressing the ball outward, stretching your arms, and releasing tension. Repeat the movement, concentrating on the sensation of energy flowing through your body.

Tree Pose (3 min)

Stand tall, feet hip-width apart. Shift your weight to one foot and lift the other off the ground, pressing the sole against the inner thigh or calf of the standing leg. Bring your palms together at your heart's center, lengthen your spine, and cast a soft gaze ahead. Consider yourself a strong tree with deep roots in the ground. Hold for a few breaths and then switch sides. This pose improves balance, concentration, and grounding.

CHAPTER 3

GENTLE JOINT MOBILITY FOR SENIORS

Gentle joint mobilization is an important part of Tai Chi practice for elders. These exercises increase flexibility, range of motion, and joint lubrication, resulting in more fluid and graceful Tai Chi movements.

Warm-up (Before starting)

Neck Rolls
Slowly move your head in a circular motion, forward and backward, a few times in each direction.

Shoulder Rolls

Gently roll your shoulders forward and backward a few times.

Wrist Circles
Draw small circles forward and backward a few times in each direction.

Ankle Circles
Rotate your ankles slowly clockwise and counterclockwise a few times in each direction.

Exercises For Joint Mobilization

Slanted Head
Place your feet shoulder-width apart and incline your knees slightly. Without straining, slowly bend your head to one side and bring your ear close to your shoulder. Hold on for a brief while.

On the other side, repeat. On both sides, repeat this motion numerous times.

Arm Circles
Bend your knees slightly and place your feet shoulder-width apart.
Spread your arms out to the sides, palms down.
Repeatedly move your arms forward in tiny, deliberate circles.
Turn around and make a few little circles go backward.
Steer clear of jerky movements and maintain a calm posture.

Mild Twists
Place your feet shoulder-width apart and incline your knees slightly.
Maintaining your feet firmly planted, carefully rotate your upper body from side to side,focusing on the way your

spine rotates. Look over your shoulder
to twist without putting too much
strain on your neck. Do this movement
a few times in each direction, moving
slowly and carefully each time.

Swinging legs
Maintain a straight leg and an engaged
core as you swing one leg forward and
backward several times.
Stand with your feet shoulder-width
apart and prop yourself up against a
chair or wall.
Continue with the opposite leg.
Steer clear of big swings and
concentrate on deliberate motions.

Bends In The Ankles
Place your feet shoulder-width apart
and, if needed, grasp onto a solid chair
or wall for stability. Repeat with the
opposite leg. Slowly shift your weight

to one leg and bend the ankle of the leg
that is standing, pointing your toes up
and down a few times.
Repeat on the other leg.
Keep your movements under control
and avoid excessive bouncing.

STRETCHING FOR FLEXIBILITY

Stretching is a vital component of Tai Chi, especially for seniors. It helps improve flexibility, reduce muscle stiffness, and enhance the overall effectiveness of the practice. When seated, these stretches are safe and accessible, providing numerous benefits without putting undue strain on the body.

Neck Stretches

Side-To-Side Stretch (1-2 minutes)
Sit upright with your feet flat on the ground and hands resting on your thighs.

Slowly tilt your head to the right, bringing your right ear towards your right shoulder. Hold for 15-20 seconds. Slowly tilt your head to the left, bringing your left ear towards your left shoulder. Hold for 15-20 seconds.

Forward And Backward Stretch (1-2 minutes)

Sit upright with your feet flat on the ground and hands resting on your thighs.

Gently lower your chin towards your chest, feeling the stretch along the back of your neck. Hold for 15-20 seconds.

Lift your chin slightly and tilt your head back gently, feeling the stretch along the front of your neck. Hold for 15-20 seconds.

Shoulder And Arm Stretches

Shoulder Rolls (1-2 minutes)

Sit upright with your feet flat on the ground and hands resting on your thighs.

Lift your shoulders up towards your ears, roll them back, and then down. Perform this movement slowly and smoothly.

Reverse the direction by rolling your shoulders forward.

Overhead Stretch (1-2 minutes)

Sit upright with your feet flat on the ground.

Extend your arms overhead, interlock your fingers, and turn your palms upward. Hold this stretch for 15-20 seconds.

This stretch elongates the spine and stretches the shoulders and upper back.

Torso And Spine Stretches

Seated Spinal Twist (2-3 minutes)
Sit upright with your feet flat on the
ground.
Place your right hand on the outside of
your left thigh and your left hand
behind you on the chair. Gently twist
your torso to the left, looking over
your left shoulder. Hold for 15-20
seconds.
Switch sides by placing your left hand
on the outside of your right thigh and
your right hand behind you on the
chair. Twist to the right and hold for
15-20 seconds.

Side Stretch (1-2 minutes)
Sit upright with your feet flat on the
ground.
Raise your right arm overhead and
gently lean to the left, feeling the

stretch along the right side of your
body. Hold for 15-20 seconds.
Raise your left arm overhead and lean
to the right, holding for 15-20 seconds.

Leg And Hip Stretches

Hamstring Stretch (1-2 minutes)

Sit at the edge of your chair with one
leg extended straight out in front of
you, heel on the floor.
Keep your back straight and hinge
forward at the hips, reaching towards
your toes. Hold for 15-20 seconds.
Switch legs and repeat the stretch.

Hip Opener (1-2 minutes)

Sit upright with your feet flat on the
ground.
Lift your right ankle and place it on
your left knee. Gently press down on

your right knee, feeling the stretch in your hip. Hold for 15-20 seconds. Switch legs and repeat the stretch.

Ankle And Foot Stretches

Ankle Circles (1-2 minutes)

Sit upright with your feet flat on the ground.

Lift one foot off the ground and rotate your ankle in slow circles. Perform 10 circles in each direction.

Switch to the other foot and repeat the circles.

Toe Flex And Point (1-2 minutes)

Sit upright with your feet flat on the ground.

Lift one foot off the ground, flex your toes up towards your shin, and then point them down towards the floor. Repeat this movement 10 times.

Switch to the other foot and repeat the stretch.

CHAPTER 4

SEATED TAI CHI MOVEMENTS

Seated warm-up exercises are essential for preparing the body and mind for Tai Chi practice, especially for the elderly.

Neck Rolls (1-2 minutes)
Sit comfortably, back straight, shoulders relaxed. Gently lower your chin to your chest, then slowly roll your head to the right, bringing your right ear near your right shoulder. Hold for a few seconds before rolling your head back to center and repeating on the left side. Continue to alternate sides, moving slowly and mindfully.

Shoulder Rolls (1-2 minutes)

Sit tall and relax your arms at your sides. Inhale as you raise your shoulders to your ears, then exhale as you roll them back and forth in a circular motion.

Repeat this movement several times, then switch directions, rolling your shoulders forward before lifting them up and backward.

Arm Circles (1-2 minutes)

Extend your arms out to the sides at shoulder level, palms down. Inhale as you circle your arms forward and bring your fingertips together at the front of your body. Exhale as you continue the circle, bringing your arms out to the sides and then back behind you.

Repeat this movement several times, then switch directions.

Spinal Twists (1-2 minutes)

Sit upright with your feet flat on the ground and your hands resting on your knees. Inhale to lengthen your spine, then exhale to twist your torso to the right, resting your left hand on your right knee and your right hand behind you for support. Hold for a few breaths, then inhale as you return to the center. Repeat on the left side.

Ankle Circles (1-2 minutes)
Sit tall, feet flat on the floor. Extend your right leg in front of you and circle your ankle clockwise, then counterclockwise. Repeat this movement a few times before switching legs and repeating on the left side.

CORE-SEATED TAI CHI MOVEMENTS FOR SENIORS

Prepare For Practice (1-2 minutes)
Choose a quiet, comfortable space to practice seated Tai Chi.
Sit up straight in a sturdy chair, feet flat on the floor and hands comfortably resting on your thighs or knees.

Centering Breath (1 minute)
Close your eyes gently and breathe deeply through your nose, allowing your abdomen to expand.
Take a slow and complete exhale through your mouth, releasing any tension or stress with each breath.

Alignment And Relaxation (1 minute)
Gently lengthen your spine, stacking each vertebra on top of the other.

Relax your shoulders away from your
ears.

Relax your facial muscles, jaw, and
forehead, allowing your body to settle
into a relaxed yet alert position.

Begin Cloud Hands (3-5 minutes)
Position your arms in front of your body, palms facing each other.
Shift your weight to your left foot while rotating your torso to the left, allowing your right hand to float up and your left hand to drift down.
Reverse the movement, shifting your weight to your right foot and rotating your torso to the right, allowing your left hand to rise while your right hand falls.
Continue this flowing movement, synchronized with your breath.
Imagine your hands tracing clouds in the sky as you move around.
Slow down the movement and bring your hands to rest at your sides.

Seated Tai Chi, Embracing The Tree(3-5 minutes)

Place your hands on your chest with palms facing inward.

Slowly open your arms to the sides, as if to embrace a tree.

Return your hands to your chest, repeating the motion.

Concentrate on the gentle opening and closing of the chest.

Seated Tai Chi Swaying Willow
(3-5 minutes)

Sit comfortably, hands on lap.
Inhale and raise one arm overhead,
leaning slightly to the opposite side.
Exhale, bring the arm back down, and
repeat on the opposite side.
Imagine a willow tree swaying with
each movement.

Seated Tai Chi Floating Clouds
(2-3 minutes)
Inhale while lifting both arms
overhead, palms facing each other.
Exhale as you lower your arms back
into your lap.
Imagine the gentle movement of
clouds floating in the sky.
Concentrate on smooth, continuous
motion.

**Seated Tai Chi Gentle Twist
(2-3 minutes)**

Sit with your back straight and your
hands in your lap.
Inhale and twist your upper body to
one side.
Exhale, return to the centre, and repeat
on the opposite side.
Keep your movements slow and
controlled.

**Seated Tai Chi Cloud Hands
(2-3 minutes)**

Begin with your hands in front of your chest, palms facing downward.
In a circular motion, raise one hand and lower the other.
Imagine gently guiding clouds with your hands.
Coordinate the movement with your breath to create a continuous flow.

Seated Tai Chi Floating Butterfly(2-3 minutes)

Place your hands on your lap with palms facing each other.
Inhale while lifting one hand up, fingers fluttering like butterflies.
Exhale and lower the hand back to your lap, then repeat with the other hand.

Seated Tai Chi Rocking Boat(2-3 minutes)

Sit with your back straight and feet flat on the floor.
Hold on to the sides of your chair for stability.
Inhale while leaning back slightly.
Exhale and return to an upright position.

Seated Tai Chi With Harmonious Breathing(2-3 minutes)

Place one hand on your chest, the other on your abdomen.
Inhale deeply, expanding your abdomen first, then your chest.
Exhale slowly, first from your chest, then from your abdomen.
Concentrate on the rhythmic rise and fall of your hands in time with your breath.

Seated Tai Chi Cloud Hands Variation(2-3 minutes)

Hold your hands in front of your chest, palms up.
Rotate your hands in a circular motion to form small circles.
Reverse the directions of the circles.

Seated Tai Chi Gentle Head Tilt
(2-3 minutes)

Sit with your back straight and hands
on your lap.
Inhale while tilting your head to one
side, ear to shoulder.
Exhale, return to the centre, and repeat
on the opposite side.
Maintain a gentle, controlled
movement.

Seated Tai Chi Rising Sun(2-3
minutes)

Sit with your back straight and your
hands in your lap.
Inhale, extend your arms forward, and
raise your gaze.
Exhale, lowering your arms and eyes.

Consider the rising sun as you raise
your arms, and the soothing descent as
you lower them.

Seated Tai Chi Healing Waves
(2-3 minutes)

Extend both arms forward, palms
facing downward.
Inhale and lift your arms in a
wave-like motion.
Exhale, lowering your arms in a
flowing motion.
Consider the soothing waves of the
ocean.

Seated Tai Chi Lotus Blossom(2-3
minutes)

Rest your hands on your lap, palms up.
Inhale as you spread your hands
outward, picturing a lotus blossom
blooming.
Exhale and bring your hands together
in a gentle closing motion.

Connect to the image of a serene lotus opening and closing.

Seated Tai Chi Calming Waves(2-3 minutes)

Place your hands on your lap with palms facing down.
Inhale, lift one hand, and imagine a wave rising.
Exhale, lower your hand, and imagine the wave gently returning to the ocean.
Repeat with the other hand to create a rhythmic, relaxing flow.

Seated Tai Chi, Flowing River(2-3 minutes)

Extend your arms forward, palms facing downward.
Inhale and move your arms in a flowing, undulating motion.
Exhale and continue the river-like movement.

Imagine your arms as a gentle river meandering.

Seated Tai Chi Mountain Pose(2-3 minutes)

Sit with your back straight and your hands in your lap.
Inhale and raise both arms overhead, gently stretching.
Exhale, lowering your hands, feeling rooted like a mountain.
Connect with the stability and strength of the mountain.

Seated Tai Chi Wisdom Tree(2-3 minutes)

Place one hand on your abdomen, the other on your heart.
Inhale and imagine energy rising from your abdomen to your heart.

Exhale and feel the flow of wisdom
and tranquillity.
Concentrate on the symbiotic
relationship between your abdomen
and heart.

Seated Tai Chi Gentle Breeze(2-3 minutes)

Position your hands in front of your chest, palms facing each other.
Inhale as you separate your hands, feeling a gentle breeze.
Exhale, bringing your hands back together and enjoying the soothing breeze
Visualize the gentle and relaxing movement of air.

Seated Tai Chi Oceanic Breath(2-3 minutes)

Inhale deeply through your nose, imagining waves filling your lungs.
Exhale slowly through your mouth, imagining the waves receding.
Connect your breath to the ocean's natural rhythms.

Cultivate a sense of calm with each
breath.

Seated Tai Chi Gratitude Gesture(2-3 minutes)

Place your hands on your heart in a
prayer-like position.
Inhale and express gratitude for the
good things in your life.
Exhale to relieve any tension or
worries.
Focus on the warmth and appreciation
within your heart.

Seated Tai Chi Gentle Twist And Reach(2-3 minutes)

Sit with your back straight and hands
on your lap.
Inhale and twist your upper body to
one side.
Exhale, reaching towards the opposite
side.

Feel the gentle stretch and rotation through your spine.

Seated Tai Chi Unity Flow(2-3 minutes)

Interlace your fingers, palms facing out.
Inhale, extend your arms forward, creating a sense of unity.
Exhale, bringing your hands back to your lap, feeling centered and connected.
Embrace the idea of unity within yourself and with the world.

Seated Tai Chi Butterfly Wings(2-3 minutes)

Place your hands on your lap with palms facing each other.
Inhale and spread your hands like butterfly wings.

Exhale and bring your hands back together.
Repeat for 2-3 minutes, focusing on gentle, fluttering movements.

Seated Tai Chi with Waving Leaves(2-3 minutes)

Extend one arm diagonally overhead, fingers resembling leaves.
Inhale, imagining the leaves reaching for the sun.
Exhale and gracefully lower your arm.
Repeat for 1-2 minutes on each side, keeping a smooth rhythm.

Seated Tai Chi Radiant Sunflower(3-5 minutes)

Interlace your fingers and lift your arms up.
Inhale and reach for the sky like a sunflower.

Exhale and bring your arms back
down.

Seated Tai Chi Crescent Moon(2-3 minutes)

Inhale and lift one arm overhead in a crescent shape.
Exhale and lean gently to the opposite side.
Repeat for 1-2 minutes on each side, focusing on the elongation of the spine.

Seated Tai Chi Ripple Effect

Place your hands on your lap with palms facing down.
Inhale, making a ripple-like motion with your arms.
Exhale, allowing the ripple to flow back.
Repeat for 2-3 minutes, focusing on smooth, continuous movement.

Seated Tai Chi Wisdom Owl

Slowly rotate your head to look over your shoulder.
Inhale while turning, then exhale as you return to the center.
Repeat for 1-2 minutes on each side to increase neck flexibility.

Seated Tai Chi Gentle Dragon
Inhale and raise both arms forward and upward.
Exhale and lower your arms in a graceful, dragon-like motion.
Repeat for 3-4 minutes, channeling the spirit of a gentle dragon.

Seated Tai Chi, Tranquil Lake
Inhale deeply and expand your chest.
Exhale slowly, picturing ripples on a tranquil lake.
Repeat for 3-5 minutes, synchronizing your breathing to the imagery.

Seated Taichi Harmony Windmill

Extend your arms to the sides, shoulder height.
Inhale and rotate your arms in a windmill motion.
Exhale and continue the circular movement.
Repeat for 2-3 minutes to create a sense of harmony.

Seated Tai Chi Infinite Infinity

Inhale and draw an infinity symbol with your hands.
Exhale and allow the symbol to expand and contract.
Repeat for 3-5 minutes to connect with the infinite flow of energy.

Seated Tai Chi Cloud Dragons

Inhale and lift one arm in a swirling motion.

Exhale and guide the imaginary cloud dragon with your hand.
Repeat for 2-3 minutes on each side, enjoying the cloud dragons' dance.

Seated Tai Chi, Gentle Swaying Bamboo

Place your hands in front of your chest with palms facing each other.
Inhale deeply, imagining your arms as supple bamboo swaying in the breeze.
Exhale and move with a gentle sway.
Repeat for 3-4 minutes to help bamboo become more flexible.

Seated Tai Chi Moonlit Reflection

Extend one leg forward, toes pointed up.
Inhale, bringing your hands to your toes.
Exhale and fold forward with a gentle stretch.

Repeat for 1-2 minutes on each leg, concentrating on the reflection-like movement.

Seated Tai Chi Flowing Koi Fish
Inhale and extend one arm forward and
the opposite leg.
Exhale and return to the starting
position.
Repeat for 2-3 minutes on each side,
capturing the fluidity of a koi fish.

Seated Tai Chi, Gentle Crane
Inhale, extend one leg forward, and
raise your arms.
Exhale, lowering your leg and arms
gracefully.
Repeat for 2-3 minutes on each side to
capture the gracefulness of a crane.

**Seated Tai Chi, Tranquil Lake
Reflection**
Inhale and raise your arms overhead.
Exhale and lean gently to one side,
creating a lake-like reflection.

Repeat for 1-2 minutes on each side, finding peace in the movement.

Seated Tai Chi With Fluttering Leaves

Inhale and extend your arms to the sides.
Exhale and flutter your fingers.
Repeat for 3-4 minutes, enjoying the lightness of the fluttering leaves.

Seated Tai Chi, Peaceful Swan

Inhale, extend one leg diagonally, and raise your arms.
Exhale, lowering your leg and arms gracefully.
Repeat for 2-3 minute

Fair Lady Works At Shuttles

Sit on a sturdy chair with your feet flat on the ground and your back supported.

Begin by sitting upright with your spine straight and your shoulders relaxed.

Place your hands on your thighs or knees, palms facing down, and take a deep breath in.

Exhale as you lean slightly to the left side, allowing your left hand to slide down your left leg towards your knee while reaching your right arm up and over towards the left side.

Continue this gentle rocking motion from side to side, coordinating your movements with your breath.

Repeat for 2-3 Minutes

Embrace Tiger, Return To Mountain

Sit on a sturdy chair with your feet flat on the ground and your back supported.

Begin by sitting upright with your spine straight and your shoulders relaxed.

Place your hands on your thighs or knees, palms facing down, and take a deep breath in.

Gently lean forward from your hips, bringing your torso towards your thighs while allowing your arms to hang loosely towards the ground, as if embracing a tiger.

Keep your spine long and your neck relaxed, allowing your head to hang naturally.

Repeat the movement, this time gently leaning back from your hips, allowing your chest to open and your arms to

extend out to the sides, as if returning
to the mountain.
Repeat 3-5 minutes

High Pat On Horse(3-5Minutes)

Begin by sitting upright with your spine straight and your shoulders relaxed.

Lift your right hand up towards your right shoulder, palm facing down, as if you are patting a horse's back.

At the same time, extend your left arm out to the side at shoulder height, palm facing down, as if reaching out to guide the horse.

Slowly switch sides by lowering your right hand back down to your side and lifting your left hand up towards your left shoulder, palm facing down.

At the same time, extend your right arm out to the side at shoulder height, palm facing down, as if reaching out with your other hand to guide the horse.

Carry Tiger To Mountain(3-5 Minutes)

Sit upright with your spine straight and your shoulders relaxed.
Extend your arms out to the sides at shoulder height, palms facing down, as if you are about to embrace a large ball.
Inhale deeply as you twist your torso to the left, bringing your right hand across your body towards your left side while keeping your left arm extended out to the side.
Exhale slowly as you return to the center and twist your torso to the right, bringing your left hand across your body towards your right side while keeping your right arm extended out to the side.

Imagine as if you are carrying a tiger
across the mountain, moving with
strength and fluidity.
Continue to flow smoothly from one
side to the other, coordinating your
movements with your breath.
Keep your movements fluid and
controlled, allowing your breath to
guide the rhythm of the exercise.

White Stork Spreads Wings(3-5 Minutes)

Sit upright with your spine straight and your shoulders relaxed.

Raise your arms out to the sides at shoulder height, palms facing down, like the wings of a white stork spreading wide.

Exhale slowly as you lower your arms back down to your sides, maintaining a gentle and controlled movement.

Inhale deeply as you once again raise your arms out to the sides at shoulder height, palms facing down.

Lower your arms back down to your sides, maintaining a smooth and fluid motion.

Repeat this movement several times, syncing your breath with the movement of your arms.

Needle At Sea Bottom(3-5 Minutes)

Shift your weight slightly to one side
while maintaining your balance.
Lift one foot off the ground and extend
it forward, keeping your knee slightly
bent and your toes pointed.
Imagine you are lowering a needle
gently towards the sea bottom,
maintaining a sense of fluidity and
grace in your movement.
Shift your weight to the opposite side
and lift your other foot off the ground,
extending it forward in a controlled
manner.
Continue to visualize the gentle
descent of the needle towards the sea
bottom, maintaining smooth and
steady movements.

Punch Downward(3-5 Minutes)

Raise your right arm to shoulder
height, keeping your elbow slightly
bent and your fist closed.
Extend your arm downward in a
punching motion, aiming towards the
ground with controlled force.
Slowly return your arm to the starting
position, maintaining a steady and
controlled movement.
Raise your left arm to shoulder height,
keeping your elbow slightly bent and
your fist closed.
Inhale deeply as you extend your left
arm downward in a punching motion,
mirroring the movement of your right
arm.
Exhale slowly as you return your left
arm to the starting position,
maintaining control and balance.

Withdraw And Push(3-5minutes)

Sit comfortably on a sturdy chair with your feet flat on the ground and your back straight.
Place your hands on your thighs or knees, palms facing down, and take a few deep breaths to center yourself.
Place your hands in front of you at chest height, palms facing each other about shoulder-width pull your hands back towards your chest, bending your elbows.
Imagine gathering energy towards your center as you withdraw your hands.
Visualize pushing away any tension or negative energy, maintaining a steady and controlled motion.
Inhale as you withdraw your hands towards your chest, and exhale as you push them forward.

Gradually slow down the movement,
bringing your hands back to rest on
your thighs.

Cross Hands(3-5 minutes)

Sit comfortably on a sturdy chair with your feet flat on the ground and your back straight.
Place your hands on your thighs or knees, palms facing down, and take a few deep breaths to center yourself.
Lift your arms in front of you, bringing them up to chest height with palms facing inward.
Cross your wrists in front of your chest, with one hand over the other, forming an "X" shape.
Choose a hand to be on top, and then switch in subsequent repetitions.
Exhale slowly as you uncross your wrists and lower your hands back down to your thighs in a controlled manner.

Part The Horse's Mane

Sit comfortably on a sturdy chair with your feet flat on the ground and your back straight.
Place your hands on your thighs or knees, palms facing down, and take a few deep breaths to center yourself.
Begin with your hands in front of you at chest height, palms facing each other as if holding a small ball.
Move your right hand downward and backward, palm facing down, as if smoothing the horse's mane.
Exhale slowly as you bring your hands back to the starting position, forming the ball again in front of your chest.
Exhale slowly as you return to the starting position.
Repeat For 3-5 minutes

CHAPTER 5

ADDRESSING ARTHRITIS AND JOINT PAIN

Arthritis and joint pain are common concerns for seniors, often leading to reduced mobility and a decrease in the quality of life. However, seated Tai Chi offers a gentle yet effective way to manage these issues, providing relief and improving overall well-being. Here's how seated Tai Chi can help address arthritis and joint pain for seniors.

Low-Impact Exercises
Seated Tai Chi involves slow, controlled movements that are easy on the joints. Unlike high-impact exercises, these movements do not strain the joints, making it suitable for those with arthritis.
The flowing movements of Tai Chi help maintain and improve the range of motion in

the joints. Regular practice can prevent
stiffness and enhance flexibility, which is
crucial for those with arthritis.

Improved Circulation

Tai Chi promotes better blood circulation
throughout the body. Improved circulation
helps reduce inflammation and delivers
essential nutrients to the joints, aiding in
pain relief and joint health.
The gentle movements and rhythmic
breathing in Tai Chi stimulate the body's
natural pain-relieving mechanisms. Over
time, this can lead to a reduction in chronic
pain associated with arthritis.

Muscle Strengthening

Tai Chi strengthens the muscles around the
joints, providing better support and stability.
Stronger muscles can reduce the load on the
joints, alleviating pain and preventing
further damage.
Seated Tai Chi also focuses on core strength,
which is vital for overall stability and
balance. A strong core helps in maintaining

proper posture and reduces the risk of falls, which is particularly important for seniors.

Flexibility

Regular practice of Tai Chi helps improve flexibility in the muscles and joints. Increased flexibility can lead to better mobility and a greater ability to perform daily activities with ease.

Tai Chi enhances balance and coordination, which are often compromised in individuals with arthritis. Improved balance reduces the risk of falls and injuries, contributing to overall joint health.

Stress Reduction

Tai Chi incorporates deep breathing and mindfulness, which help reduce stress and anxiety. Stress can exacerbate pain and inflammation, so managing stress is crucial for those with arthritis.

Tai Chi promotes a strong mind-body connection, fostering a sense of control and well-being. This connection can empower individuals to manage their symptoms more effectively and improve their quality of life.

Seated Wave Hands Like Clouds
(Duration: 2-3 minutes)
Sit upright with your feet flat on the ground and hands resting on your thighs.
Slowly lift both arms in front of you to shoulder height, palms facing each other.
Gently move your arms side to side, mimicking the motion of clouds floating across the sky. Keep the movements smooth and relaxed.
Continue this movement for 2-3 minutes, focusing on the gentle flow and rhythm.

CONCLUSION

Tai Chi is more than a physical practice; it is a transformative journey that touches every aspect of our being—body, mind, and spirit. Throughout this book, we have explored how the timeless principles of Tai Chi can be harnessed to restore and enhance balance, build resilience, and cultivate a deep sense of inner peace. Whether you are seeking improved physical stability, mental clarity, or emotional calm, Tai Chi offers a path to achieve these goals with grace and mindfulness.

For those on the journey of aging, recovery, or simply seeking a more balanced life, Tai Chi serves as a powerful tool to keep the body agile, the mind sharp, and the spirit centered.

By integrating the practices of grounding, centering, and mindful movement, you unlock the potential for greater vitality, strength, and equilibrium, no matter where you are in life. The slow, flowing movements are not just exercises—they are a profound expression of connection to the earth, to your body, and to the rhythm of life itself.

Remember that balance is not a destination, but a continuous process. It is something that evolves with each breath, each movement, and each moment of mindfulness. The benefits of Tai Chi extend far beyond the physical realm—improving your overall quality of life, enhancing your energy levels, and fostering a sense of harmony that flows into every aspect of your daily experience.

As you continue your Tai Chi practice,
let it be a reminder that balance is an
ongoing journey, one that can be
embraced at any age or stage of life.
With patience, consistency, and the
intention to stay present, you will find
that the practice of Tai Chi offers a
profound and lasting sense of
balance—both within yourself and in
the world around you.

Embrace the flow, trust the process,
and carry the calm, centered energy of
Tai Chi into every moment of your
life.